Don't Get a Menstrual Cramp

A GUIDEBOOK ON UNDERSTANDING AND SOLUTIONS TO MENSTRUAL CRAMPS

Jessica Gerald

Table of Contents

Chapter 1: What are Menstrual Cramps
Explanation of Menstrual cramps   6
Prevalence of Menstrual Cramps   8
Myths surrounding Menstrual Cramps   10
Chapter 2: Understanding Menstrual Cramps
Types of Menstrual Cramps   12
Other Causes of Menstrual Cramps   14
When to seek Medical Attention   16
Chapter 3: Managing Menstrual Cramps Naturally
Diet and Nutrition   18
Exercise and Physical Activity   20
Heat Therapy   22
Herbal Remedies and Supplements   24
Acupuncture and Massage   25
Chapter 4: Medical Treatment for Menstrual Cramps
Over-the-Counter Pain Relievers   26
Prescription Medications   28
Hormonal Birth Control   30
Surgical Procedures   32
Chapter 5: Lifestyle Changes to Prevent Menstrual Cramps
Maintaining a Healthy Weight   33
Getting Enough Sleep   35
Maintaining Good Hygiene   37
Chapter 6: Alternative and Complementary Treatments
Chiropractic Care   41
Homeopathy   43
Ayurvedic Medicine   45
Naturopathic Medicine   47
Chapter 7:Conclusion
Recap of Menstrual Cramps and their Management   49
Final Thoughts and Encouragement to seek help if needed.   51
Additional Notes
Question Sets

Introduction

Don't Get a Menstrual Cramp is a book that aims to provide essential information and practical tips for people who experience menstrual cramps. Menstrual cramps, also known as dysmenorrhea, affect many people during their reproductive years and can be a source of discomfort and pain. This book is written with the goal of helping individuals better understand the causes of menstrual cramps and how to manage them effectively.

The book starts by explaining the menstrual cycle and the role hormones play in the process. It goes on to discuss the various types of menstrual cramps, their causes, and the symptoms that accompany them. The book also delves into the different treatment options available, both conventional and alternative, and how to implement them for maximum relief.

Don't Get a Menstrual Cramp is written in an easy-to-understand language, with practical tips and advice that readers can start implementing right away. It covers a range of topics, from lifestyle changes that can help reduce menstrual cramps to the use of pain relief medications and herbal remedies.

This book is a must-read for anyone looking to gain a better understanding of menstrual cramps and how to manage them effectively. Whether you experience mild or severe menstrual cramps, this book provides a wealth of information to help you lead a more comfortable and pain-free life.

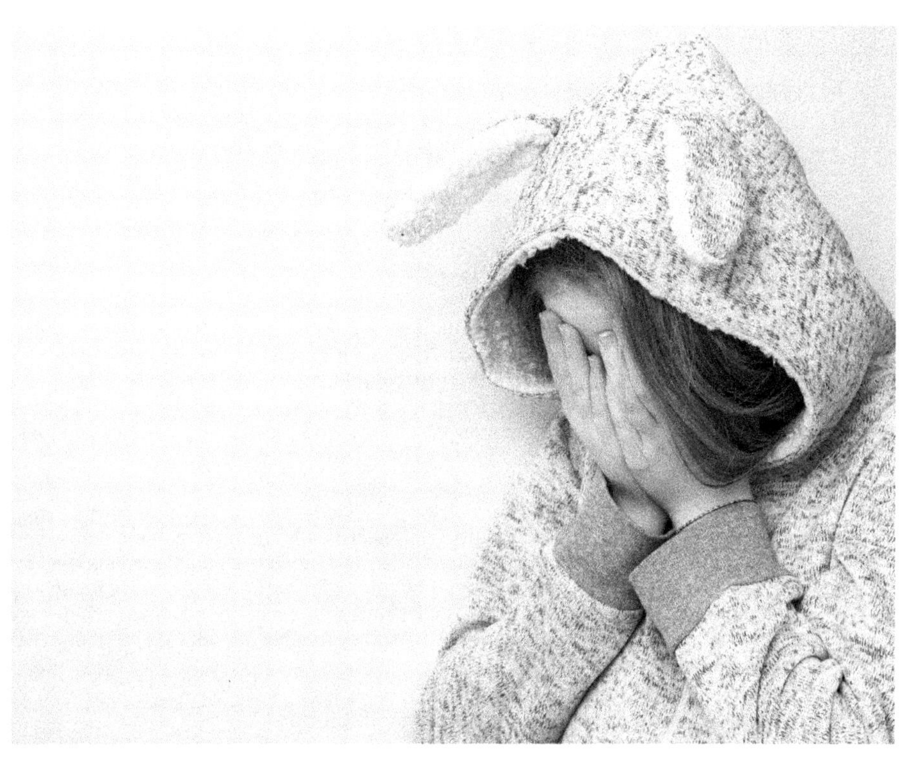

Chapter 1: What are Menstrual Cramps?

Explanation of menstrual cramps

Menstrual cramps, also known as dysmenorrhea, are a common and uncomfortable experience for many menstruating individuals. They are typically felt as pain or discomfort in the lower abdomen or pelvic region, and can range in intensity from mild to severe. Menstrual cramps usually occur just before or during menstruation, although some individuals may experience them at other times during their menstrual cycle.

Menstrual cramps are caused by the uterus contracting in order to shed its lining, which occurs during menstruation. These contractions are necessary in order for the lining to be expelled from the body, but they can also cause discomfort and pain. The severity of menstrual cramps can vary widely, and may be influenced by factors such as age, menstrual history, and individual differences in pain tolerance.

Two main types of menstrual cramps include: primary dysmenorrhea and secondary dysmenorrhea. Primary dysmenorrhea is the more common type, and is caused by the normal contractions of the uterus during menstruation. Secondary dysmenorrhea is caused by an underlying medical condition such as endometriosis or uterine fibroids. Individuals with secondary dysmenorrhea may experience more severe pain and other symptoms in addition to menstrual cramps.

Symptoms of menstrual cramps may include:

- Discomfort in the lower abdomen or pelvic area
- Cramping or spasms in the uterus
- Back pain
- Headaches
- Nausea or vomiting
- Diarrhea or constipation
- Fatigue or weakness
- Mood changes

While menstrual cramps are a normal part of the menstrual cycle for many individuals, they can be very uncomfortable and may interfere with daily activities. There are several strategies that can be used to manage menstrual cramps and reduce their severity, including:

- Buying over-the-counter pain relievers such as ibuprofen
- Getting a heating pad or hot water bottle for the lower abdomen
- Taking a warm bath or shower
- Doing mild exercises such as yoga or even stretches
- Doing relaxation techniques like deep breathing or meditation
- Getting plenty of rest and staying hydrated

In some cases, menstrual cramps may be severe enough to require medical treatment. Your healthcare provider may recommend prescription medications, such as hormonal birth control or pain relievers, or may suggest further testing to rule out any underlying medical conditions.

Overall, menstrual cramps are a common and often uncomfortable experience for many menstruating individuals. While they can be challenging to manage, there are a variety of strategies that can be used to reduce their severity and help individuals feel more comfortable during their menstrual cycle. If you are experiencing severe or persistent menstrual cramps, it is important to talk to your healthcare provider in order to rule out any underlying medical conditions and determine the best course of treatment.

Notes

Prevalence of menstrual cramps

Menstrual cramps are a prevalent condition among women of reproductive age. According to a study published in the Journal of Women's Health, approximately 84% of women experience menstrual cramps at some point in their lives. Of these, 43% reported experiencing severe cramps that interfere with their daily activities.

Another study published in the International Journal of Women's Health reported that approximately 60% of women experience menstrual cramps during their menstrual cycle. This study also found that women who experienced painful periods were more likely to experience other menstrual-related symptoms, such as bloating, fatigue, and mood changes.

Causes

As mentioned earlier, menstrual cramps occur as a result of the uterus contracting to shed its lining during menstruation. The contractions are caused by the release of prostaglandins, hormone-like substances that are produced by the lining of the uterus. Higher levels of prostaglandins can cause more intense contractions, leading to more severe menstrual cramps.

Other factors that can contribute to the prevalence of menstrual cramps include:

Age: Menstrual cramps tend to be more common among adolescent girls and young women.

Genetics: Women with a family history of menstrual cramps may be more likely to experience them.

Endometriosis: This is a condition where the tissue that normally lines the uterus grows outside of it. Women with endometriosis often experience more severe menstrual cramps.

Uterine Fibroids: These are non-cancerous growths in the uterus that can cause pain and heavy menstrual bleeding.

Pelvic Inflammatory Disease: This is an infection of the reproductive organs that can cause pain and discomfort during menstruation.

Menstrual cramps are a common condition experienced by many women. While they can be painful and uncomfortable, there are several treatments available to help manage them.

Again, If you are experiencing severe menstrual cramps, it is essential to speak with your healthcare provider to determine the underlying cause and develop an appropriate treatment plan.

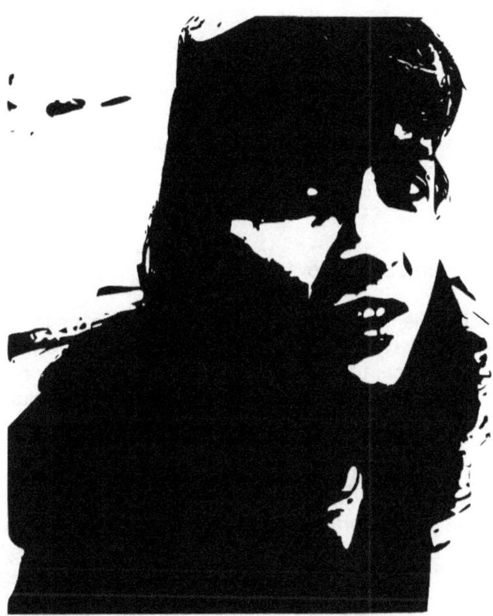

Myths surrounding Menstrual Cramps

While cramps are a natural part of the menstrual cycle, there are several myths and misconceptions surrounding them that can cause confusion and unnecessary anxiety. We'll take a closer look at some of the most common myths surrounding menstrual cramps and separate fact from fiction.

Myth #1: Menstrual cramps are not a big deal.

One of the most pervasive myths surrounding menstrual cramps is that they are not a significant issue and can be easily ignored. However, the reality is that menstrual cramps can be extremely uncomfortable and, in some cases, even debilitating. For many women, cramps can make it difficult to perform everyday activities, such as going to work or school, and can have a significant impact on their overall quality of life.

Myth #2: Menstrual cramps are caused by poor hygiene.

Another common myth surrounding menstrual cramps is that they are caused by poor hygiene or a lack of cleanliness. This is simply not true. Menstrual cramps are caused by the contractions of the uterus as it sheds its lining during menstruation. While maintaining good hygiene is important during menstruation to prevent infection, it is not a factor in the development of cramps.

Myth #3: Menstrual cramps are a sign of a serious medical condition.

While menstrual cramps can be uncomfortable and even painful, they are generally not a sign of a serious medical condition. However, in some cases, severe cramping may be a symptom of an underlying issue, such as endometriosis or uterine fibroids. If you experience unusually severe or prolonged cramping, it is important to talk to your doctor to rule out any underlying health problems.

Myth #4: Menstrual cramps can be cured by exercise.

While exercise can be beneficial for overall health and wellbeing, it is not a cure for menstrual cramps. While light exercise such as walking or yoga can help to alleviate cramping, more intense exercise can actually make cramps worse. Additionally, some women may find it difficult to exercise during menstruation due to discomfort or fatigue.

Myth #5: Menstrual cramps are the same for everyone.

While many women experience menstrual cramps, the severity and duration of cramps can vary widely from person to person. Some women may experience mild cramping that lasts only a few hours, while others may experience severe cramping that lasts for several days. The intensity and duration of cramps can also vary from one menstrual cycle to the next.

Myth #6: Menstrual cramps are only experienced by women.

While menstrual cramps are most commonly experienced by women who have a uterus, they can also be experienced by transgender men and non-binary individuals who have not undergone a hysterectomy. It is important to recognize that menstruation and menstrual cramps are not exclusive to women and that all individuals who experience them deserve access to appropriate healthcare and support.

In conclusion, menstrual cramps are a normal part of the menstrual cycle for many women, and it is important to understand the facts surrounding them. By dispelling these common myths and misconceptions, we can create a better understanding of menstrual health and support those who experience menstrual cramps. If you have concerns about your menstrual cycle or experience unusually severe cramping, be sure to talk to your doctor for personalized guidance and care.

Chapter 2: Understanding Menstrual Cramps

Types of Menstrual Cramps

Primary Dysmenorrhea

Primary Dysmenorrhea is the most common type of menstrual cramps and typically occurs in adolescents and young adults. It is caused by the contraction of the uterus as it sheds its lining during menstruation. Prostaglandins, hormone-like substances produced by the uterus, are responsible for these contractions. Higher levels of prostaglandins can cause more severe cramps. Symptoms of primary dysmenorrhea typically begin a few hours before menstruation and last for 2-3 days.

- Symptoms can include:
- Cramping pain in the lower abdomen and back
- Nausea and vomiting
- Diarrhea or constipation
- Headaches
- Dizziness etc

Primary dysmenorrhea is often manageable with over-the-counter pain relievers such as ibuprofen or naproxen. Other self-care measures include exercise, heat therapy, and relaxation techniques.

Secondary Dysmenorrhea

Secondary Dysmenorrhea occurs due to an underlying medical condition that affects the reproductive system. It can develop at any age, but it is more common in people in their 30s and 40s. Conditions that can cause secondary dysmenorrhea include:

- ❖ Endometriosis: A condition in which tissue similar to the lining of the uterus grows outside the uterus.
- ❖ Adenomyosis: A condition in which the tissue that lines the uterus grows into the muscular wall of the uterus.
- ❖ Fibroids: Noncancerous growths in the uterus.
- ❖ Pelvic Inflammatory Disease (PID): An infection of the reproductive organs.

Symptoms of secondary dysmenorrhea can be similar to primary dysmenorrhea but may last longer and be more severe. Treatment for secondary dysmenorrhea will depend on the underlying condition and may include medication, surgery, or other treatments.

Ovulatory Cramps
Ovulation cramps occur when an egg is released from the ovary during ovulation. It can cause mild to moderate pain in the lower abdomen, usually on one side. Ovulatory cramps can be mistaken for menstrual cramps, but they occur mid-cycle and last only a few hours to a day.

Mid-cycle Cramps
Mid-cycle cramps can occur during ovulation or can be caused by conditions such as ovarian cysts or fibroids. These cramps can range from mild to severe and can last for a few hours to a few days.

Prostaglandin-associated Syndrome (PMS)
Some people with menstruation experience a group of symptoms known as prostaglandin-associated syndrome (PMS). It can include cramps, as well as other symptoms such as mood changes, breast tenderness, and bloating.

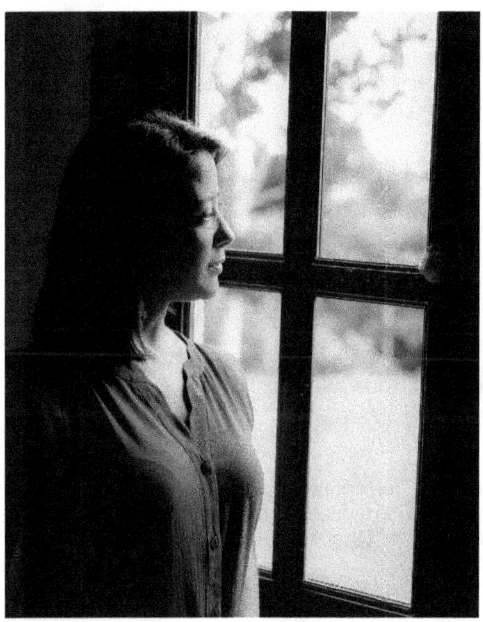

Other Causes of Menstrual Cramps

Ovarian Cysts

They are sacs filled with fluid that develop in the ovaries, which are part of the female reproductive system. They can cause pain and discomfort, including severe menstrual cramps.

They are usually benign and cause no symptoms. However, some cysts can grow large and cause pain, bloating, or other symptoms. In uncommon cases, ovarian cysts can be cancerous.

There are several types of ovarian cysts, including functional cysts, which form during ovulation and usually go away on their own; dermoid cysts, which contain tissue from other parts of the body and can cause pain; and cystadenomas, which are filled with a watery or mucous-like substance and can grow very large.

Cervical Stenosis

Cervical stenosis is a condition where the opening of the cervix is narrow, which can lead to menstrual cramps. When the cervix is narrow, it can make it difficult for the menstrual blood to flow out, which can cause the uterus to contract more forcefully, leading to more severe cramps.

In some cases, cervical stenosis can also cause an obstruction in the flow of menstrual blood, leading to painful periods and even the formation of blood clots.

Intrauterine device (IUD)

Some women may experience menstrual cramps after getting an IUD, which is a form of birth control that is inserted into the uterus. The cramps may be caused by the presence of the IUD itself, which can cause the uterus to contract.

Additionally, hormonal IUDs contain a progestin hormone, which can cause changes to the lining of the uterus and affect menstrual flow.

Stress

Stress can affect hormone levels and contribute to menstrual cramps. When you experience stress, your body releases hormones such as cortisol and adrenaline. These hormones can affect the levels of other hormones in your body, including those that regulate your menstrual cycle.

Stress can also cause your muscles to tighten, which can increase the severity of menstrual cramps. In addition, stress can make it more difficult for you to relax and can increase your sensitivity to pain, making the cramps feel more intense.

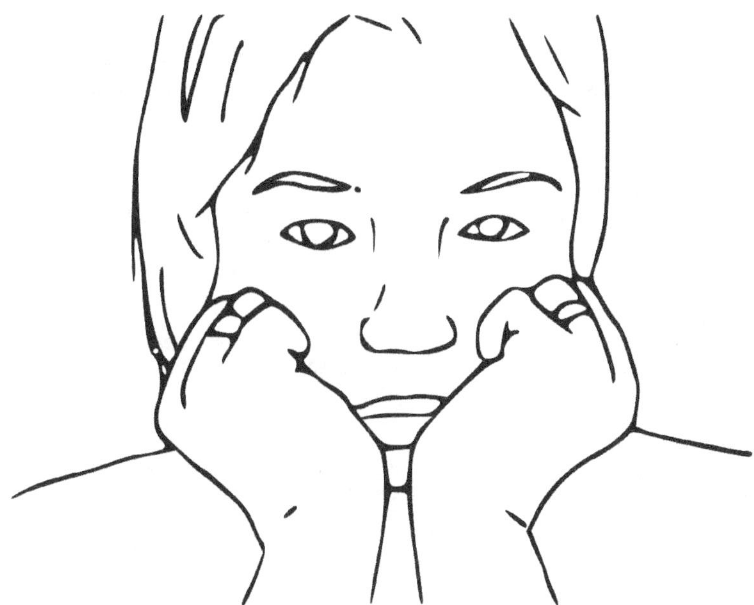

When to seek Medical Attention

Severe or persistent menstrual cramps may indicate an underlying health issue that requires medical attention. Here are some guidelines for when to seek medical attention for menstrual cramps:

Severe Pain

If your menstrual cramps are severe enough to disrupt your daily activities or require you to take painkillers frequently, it may be a sign of an underlying medical condition.

Longer than Usual

If your menstrual cramps last longer than usual or start earlier than expected in your menstrual cycle, it could be a sign of an underlying medical condition.

Irregular Menstrual Cycle

If your menstrual cycle is irregular, or if you experience heavy bleeding or bleeding between periods, it could be a sign of an underlying medical condition.

Age

If you are over 25 years old and experience sudden or severe menstrual cramps, it could be a sign of a health issue such as endometriosis or fibroids.

Family History

If other women in your family have experienced severe menstrual cramps or have been diagnosed with endometriosis or fibroids, you may be at higher risk of developing these conditions

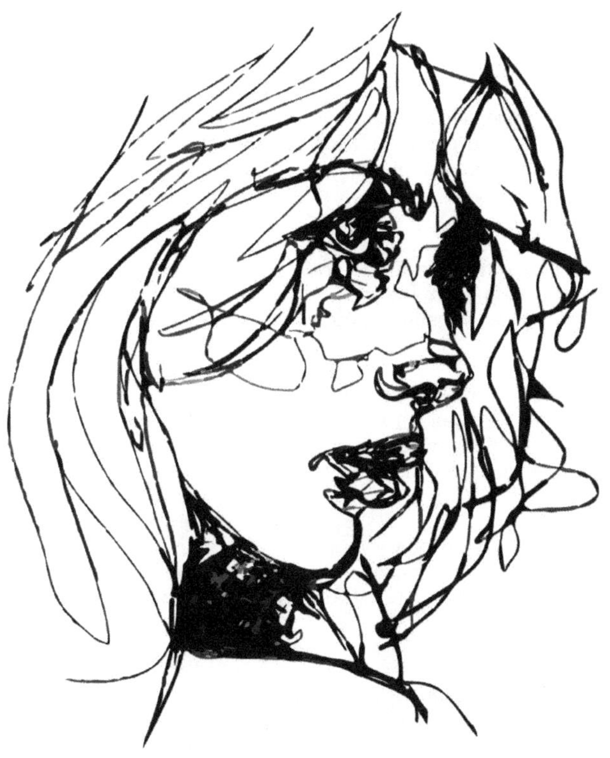

Chapter 3: Managing Menstrual Cramps Naturally

Diet and Nutrition

While over-the-counter pain medication can help alleviate some of the discomfort, a balanced diet and proper nutrition can also play a role in reducing the severity and frequency of menstrual cramps. Here are some dietary tips that may help:

Increase your intake of Magnesium-Rich Foods

Magnesium is known to help relax muscles, including the uterus. Sources of magnesium include leafy green vegetables, nuts, whole grains, and seeds.

Incorporate more Omega-3 Fatty Acids

Omega-3 fatty acids can help reduce inflammation in the body and may also help to reduce the severity of menstrual cramps. Sources of Omega-3s include fatty fish like salmon, walnuts, flaxseed and chia seeds.

Avoid Processed and High-Fat Foods

These foods can contribute to inflammation in the body and may make menstrual cramps worse. Try to avoid or limit your intake of processed foods, fried foods, and high-fat dairy products.

Include more Fruits and Vegetables in your diet

Fruits and vegetables are rich in antioxidants and other nutrients that can help reduce inflammation in the body. Aim to include a variety of colorful fruits and vegetables in your meals.

Stay Hydrated

Drinking plenty of water and other hydrating fluids can help reduce bloating and may also help to ease menstrual cramps.

Consider Herbal Remedies

Certain herbs, such as ginger, turmeric, and chamomile, have anti-inflammatory properties and may help reduce the severity of menstrual cramps. Visit your healthcare provider before trying any herbal remedies.

Overall, a balanced diet that includes plenty of nutrient-dense foods can help support overall health and may also help reduce the severity of menstrual cramps.

Notes

Exercise and Physical Activity

Exercise and physical activity can be beneficial in preventing menstrual cramps. These are some activities/exercises you can try:

Aerobic Exercise
Engaging in activities like running, brisk walking, cycling, or swimming for at least 30 minutes a day can help reduce menstrual cramps.

Yoga
Certain yoga poses can help alleviate menstrual cramps. The Cobra, Child's Pose, and Cat and Cow poses are effective for relieving cramps.

Pilates
Pilates exercises focus on strengthening the core muscles, which can help reduce menstrual cramps.

Stretching
Stretching exercises can help alleviate cramps by increasing blood flow to the muscles and reducing tension.

Dancing
Dancing is a fun and effective way to relieve menstrual cramps. It can also help improve your mood and reduce stress.

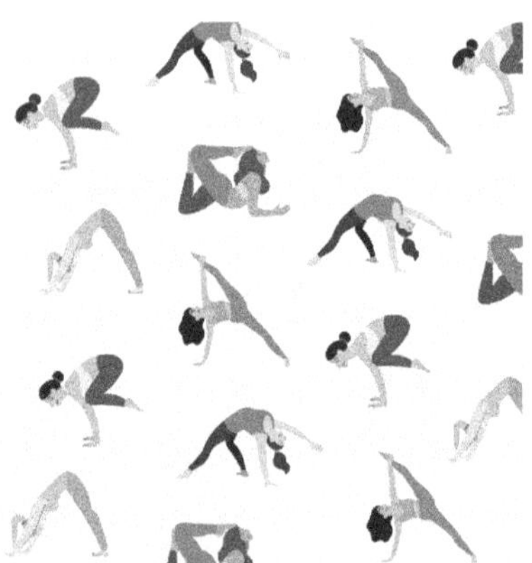

Relaxation Techniques
There are several relaxation techniques that may help alleviate menstrual cramps. Here are a few:

Deep Breathing
Deep breathing can help reduce stress and anxiety, which can contribute to menstrual cramps. Find a quiet place, sit comfortably, and breathe in through your nose for a count of four, hold for a count of four, and exhale through your mouth for a count of six.

Massage:
Gentle abdominal massage can help reduce menstrual cramps. Use circular motions with your fingers, applying a light pressure to the lower abdomen.

Warm Baths
Taking a warm bath can help relax the muscles and reduce menstrual cramps. Add some Epsom salt or essential oils like lavender to the bathwater for added relaxation.

Mindfulness Meditation
Mindfulness meditation can help reduce stress and anxiety, which can contribute to menstrual cramps. Locate a quiet place to sit comfortably, and then focus on your breath. When your mind wanders, gently bring it back to your breath.

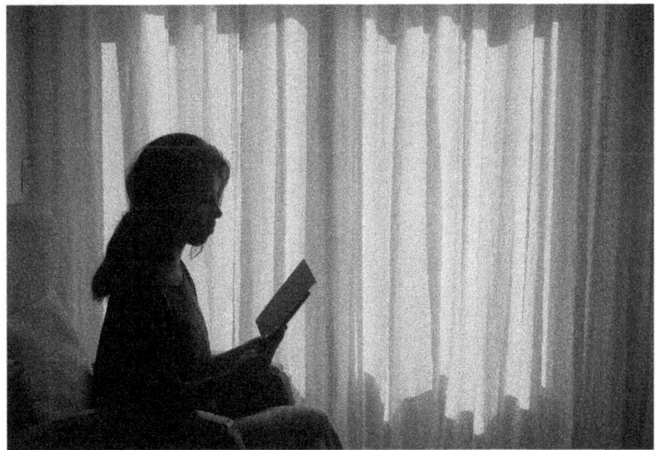

Heat Therapy

Heat therapy is a simple, natural, and effective way to relieve menstrual cramps. It works by increasing blood flow to the affected area, which helps to relax the muscles and reduce pain. There are several ways to apply heat therapy to relieve menstrual cramps, including:

Hot Water Bottle

Fill a hot water bottle with hot water and place it on your lower abdomen or lower back. The heat will help to relax the muscles and reduce the pain.

Heating Pad

Use an electric heating pad and place it on your lower abdomen or lower back. Be sure to follow the manufacturer's instructions and use the heating pad on a low or medium setup.

Warm Towel

Soak a towel in hot water, wring it out, and place it on your lower abdomen or lower back.

It's important to note that heat therapy should not be used for more than 20-30 minutes at a time. Also, be sure to use a barrier between your skin and the heat source to prevent burns.

Notes

Herbal Remedies and Supplements

Ginger
Ginger has been shown to have anti-inflammatory and pain-relieving properties, making it an effective remedy for menstrual cramps. It can be consumed in a variety of ways, including as a tea, capsule, or fresh ginger root. To make ginger tea, steep fresh ginger root in hot water for 10-15 minutes. You can also add honey or lemon for added flavor.

Turmeric
Turmeric is another spice with anti-inflammatory properties that can help alleviate menstrual cramps. It can be consumed as a spice in food or taken as a supplement in capsule form. When using turmeric as a spice, it's important to combine it with black pepper to increase its absorption.

Cinnamon
Cinnamon is a warming spice that can help increase blood flow and reduce inflammation, making it an effective natural remedy for menstrual cramps. It can be added to food or consumed as a tea by steeping cinnamon sticks in hot water for 10-15 minutes.

Chamomile
Chamomile is a natural anti-inflammatory and muscle relaxant, making it an effective remedy for menstrual cramps. It can be consumed as a tea by steeping chamomile flowers in hot water for 10-15 minutes.

Magnesium
Magnesium is a mineral that can help relax muscles and reduce inflammation, making it an effective supplement for menstrual cramps. It can be taken in capsule form or consumed through foods such as leafy green vegetables, nuts, and whole grains.

Vitamin D
Vitamin D is important for overall health and has been shown to reduce menstrual cramps. It can be consumed through foods such as fatty fish, egg yolks, and fortified dairy products, or taken as a supplement.

Omega-3 Fatty Acids
Omega-3 fatty acids are important for reducing inflammation in the body and can help alleviate menstrual cramps. They can be consumed through foods such as fatty fish, flaxseeds, and walnuts, or taken as a supplement.

Evening Primrose Oil
Evening primrose oil is a natural anti-inflammatory that can help reduce menstrual cramps. It can be taken in capsule form or added to food as a supplement.

Black Cohosh
Black cohosh is a plant that has been used for centuries to alleviate menstrual cramps. Consume as a tea or take in capsule form.

Dong Quai
Dong Quai is an herb that has been used in traditional Chinese medicine to treat menstrual cramps. Consume as a tea or take in capsule form.

While natural remedies can be effective in alleviating menstrual cramps, it's important to consult with a healthcare provider before trying any new supplements or herbs. Some herbs can interact with medications or have side effects, and it's important to ensure they are safe for you to use.

Notes

Acupuncture and Massage

Acupuncture and Massage can both be effective treatments for menstrual cramps.

Acupuncture involves the insertion of fine needles into specific points on the body, and it has been used for thousands of years to treat a variety of health conditions, including menstrual cramps. Research suggests that acupuncture can help to reduce the severity and duration of menstrual cramps by increasing blood flow to the uterus and reducing inflammation and pain.

Massage, on the other hand, involves the manipulation of the body's soft tissues, including the muscles and connective tissue. Massage can help to reduce tension and improve circulation, which can relieve menstrual cramps. Research has shown that massage therapy can be effective in reducing menstrual pain, as well as other symptoms of premenstrual syndrome (PMS).

Both acupuncture and massage are generally safe and well-tolerated, but it's always a good idea to consult with a healthcare provider before trying any new treatments, especially if you have a history of medical conditions or take any medications. It's also important to choose a qualified practitioner who has experience working with menstrual cramps and other gynecological issues.

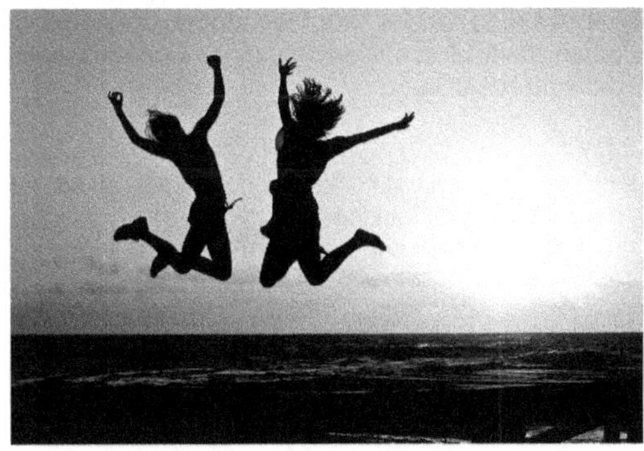

Chapter 4: Medical Treatment for Menstrual Cramps

Over-the-Counter Pain Relievers

Over-the-counter (OTC) pain relievers can be an effective way to manage menstrual cramps. We will discuss the most common OTC pain relievers for menstrual cramps.

Nonsteroidal Anti-inflammatory Drugs (NSAIDs)

NSAIDs are a type of pain reliever that works by reducing inflammation. They are the most commonly used medication for menstrual cramps. Common NSAIDs include ibuprofen, naproxen, and aspirin. These medications are available in different strengths and formulations, including tablets, capsules, and liquids.

NSAIDs work by blocking the production of prostaglandins, which are hormone-like substances that cause inflammation and pain. Prostaglandins are released in high amounts during menstruation, which is why NSAIDs are effective in managing menstrual cramps.

It is recommended to take NSAIDs before the onset of menstrual cramps, as they work better when taken early. The recommended dose of NSAIDs varies depending on the medication and strength. It is important to follow the instructions on the label or as directed by your healthcare provider.

NSAIDs can cause side effects such as stomach upset, nausea, and diarrhea. Note that It is important to take these medications with food to reduce the risk of stomach upset. People with certain medical conditions, such as kidney disease or stomach ulcers, should avoid taking NSAIDs.

Acetaminophen

Acetaminophen is another type of pain reliever that is commonly used for menstrual cramps. The way it works is by blocking pain signals in the brain. Acetaminophen is available in different strengths and formulations, including tablets, capsules, and liquids.

Acetaminophen does not have anti-inflammatory properties, so it may not be as effective as NSAIDs for managing menstrual cramps. However, it is generally considered safe and is a good alternative for people who cannot take NSAIDs due to medical conditions.

The recommended dose of acetaminophen varies depending on the strength and formulation. It is important to follow the instructions on the label or as directed by your healthcare provider. Acetaminophen can cause liver damage if taken in large amounts or for a long period of time.

Herbal Supplements
Some people may choose to use herbal supplements to manage menstrual cramps. Some herbs that have been studied for their potential to reduce menstrual cramps include ginger, cinnamon, and turmeric. However, there is limited scientific evidence to support the use of these supplements for menstrual cramps.

It is important to talk to your healthcare provider before taking any herbal supplements, as they may interact with other medications or have side effects. Some herbal supplements may also not be safe for certain populations, such as pregnant or breastfeeding women.

In conclusion, OTC pain relievers such as NSAIDs and acetaminophen can be effective in managing menstrual cramps. It is important to follow the instructions on the label or as directed by your healthcare provider. If OTC pain relievers are not effective in managing menstrual cramps, it is recommended to talk to your healthcare provider about other treatment options.

Notes

Prescription Medications

Prescription medications can be an effective treatment option for managing menstrual cramps. In this comprehensive guide, we will discuss the most commonly prescribed medications for menstrual cramps, their mechanisms of action, potential side effects, and other important considerations.

Nonsteroidal Anti-inflammatory Drugs (NSAIDs)
As mentioned earlier, NSAIDs are the most commonly prescribed medication for menstrual cramps. They work by inhibiting the production of prostaglandins, which are responsible for causing the pain and inflammation associated with menstrual cramps.

Examples of NSAIDs that are commonly prescribed for menstrual cramps include:

Ibuprofen (Advil, Motrin)
Naproxen (Aleve)
Aspirin (Bayer)
Dosage: NSAIDs should be taken as soon as cramps begin and continue for a few days, as needed. The usual dose is 200 - 400 mg every 4-6 hours.

Potential side effects: NSAIDs can cause stomach upset, nausea, vomiting, and diarrhea. They can also increase the risk of bleeding, especially if taken with other blood-thinning medications.

Hormonal Contraceptives
Hormonal Contraceptives, such as birth control pills, patches, and rings, can help reduce menstrual cramps by regulating hormone levels and reducing the amount of prostaglandins produced.

Examples of hormonal contraceptives that are commonly prescribed for menstrual cramps include:

Combined oral contraceptives (COCs), which contain both estrogen and progestin

Progestin-only contraceptives, such as the progestin-only pill, injection, implant, or IUD

Dosage: The dosage of hormonal contraceptives varies depending on the specific product and individual patient needs. It is important to consult with a healthcare provider to determine the appropriate dosage.

Potential side effects: Hormonal contraceptives can cause side effects such as nausea, headache, breast tenderness, and mood changes. They can also increase the risk of blood clots, especially in women who smoke or have other risk factors for cardiovascular disease.

Antispasmodics
Antispasmodics are medications that work by relaxing the smooth muscles in the uterus and reducing the severity of menstrual cramps.

Examples of antispasmodics that are commonly prescribed for menstrual cramps include:

Hyoscine (Scopolamine)
Dicyclomine (Bentyl)
Dosage: Antispasmodics should be taken as soon as cramps begin and continued for a few

Hormonal Birth Control

What is Hormonal Birth Control?
Hormonal Birth Control is a type of contraception that uses hormones to prevent pregnancy. There are several types of hormonal birth control available, including:

Birth Control Pills: These are pills that contain a combination of hormones (estrogen and progestin) or progestin only.

Birth Control Patch: This is a small patch that is applied to the skin and releases hormones.

Birth Control Shot: This is a shot that is given once every three months and contains progestin.

Birth Control Implant: This is a small rod that is inserted under the skin and releases hormones.

Intrauterine Device (IUD): This is a small device that is inserted into the uterus and releases hormones or copper.

How Does Hormonal Birth Control Work?
Hormonal birth control works by preventing ovulation, which is the release of an egg from the ovary. If there is no egg to fertilize, then pregnancy cannot occur. Hormonal birth control also thickens cervical mucus, making it harder for sperm to reach the egg, and thins the lining of the uterus, making it less hospitable for a fertilized egg to implant.

Benefits of Hormonal Birth Control for Menstrual Cramps
Hormonal birth control can be an effective treatment for menstrual cramps, as it can help regulate hormonal fluctuations and reduce the severity of cramps. The hormones in birth control pills, patches, and shots can reduce the amount of prostaglandins produced in the body. Prostaglandins are chemicals that cause inflammation and pain, and they are released during menstruation. By reducing the amount of prostaglandins in the body, hormonal birth control can help reduce menstrual cramps.

Additionally, hormonal birth control can help regulate menstrual cycles, which can also help reduce the severity of cramps. Birth control pills, patches, and shots can help regulate the levels of estrogen and progestin in the body, which can help reduce the fluctuations that occur during the menstrual cycle. This can lead to more predictable and less painful periods.

Potential Side Effects of Hormonal Birth Control
Like any medication, hormonal birth control can have potential side effects. Some of the most common side effects include:

- Nausea
- Headaches
- Breast tenderness
- Weight gain
- Mood changes
- Spotting or breakthrough bleeding
- Changes in libido
- Blood clots (rare)

It is important to discuss the potential risks and benefits of hormonal birth control with your healthcare provider before starting any type of contraception.

Conclusion

Hormonal birth control can be an effective treatment for menstrual cramps, as it can help regulate hormonal fluctuations and reduce the severity of cramps. However, it is important to discuss the potential risks and benefits with your healthcare provider before starting any type of contraception. If you are experiencing severe menstrual cramps, you should seek medical attention to rule out any underlying conditions.

Surgical Procedures

Primary menstrual cramps, which are caused by the uterus contracting to shed its lining during menstruation, are generally not related to surgical procedures. However, secondary menstrual cramps, which are caused by an underlying medical condition, such as endometriosis or fibroids, may require surgical intervention to treat.

In cases where the menstrual cramps are caused by an underlying medical condition, surgery may be necessary to remove the source of the pain. For example, in cases of endometriosis, surgery may be required to remove the endometrial tissue that is growing outside of the uterus and causing pain and inflammation. Similarly, in cases of fibroids, surgery may be required to remove the fibroid tumors that are causing pain and discomfort.

It is important to note that surgery is not always the first line of treatment for menstrual cramps, and that other treatments, such as hormonal contraceptives or pain relievers, may be recommended before considering surgery. Additionally, surgical procedures always carry risks and potential complications, and should only be considered after careful consideration and consultation with a healthcare provider.

After a surgical procedure, it is common for patients to experience some degree of pain and discomfort, including menstrual cramps. This is particularly true for surgeries that involve the reproductive organs, such as a hysterectomy or ovarian cyst removal. However, in most cases, the menstrual cramps that occur after surgery are temporary and can be managed with pain relievers and other self-care measures.

In summary, the relationship between menstrual cramps and surgical procedures depends on the underlying cause of the cramps. While primary menstrual cramps are generally not related to surgical procedures, secondary menstrual cramps caused by an underlying medical condition may require surgery to treat. It is important to carefully consider all treatment options and potential risks before undergoing any surgical procedure, and to follow appropriate aftercare instructions to manage any post-operative pain or discomfort, including menstrual cramps.

Chapter 5: Lifestyle Changes to Prevent Menstrual Cramps

Maintaining a Healthy Weight

One factor that can affect menstrual cramps is a woman's weight. Maintaining a healthy weight has been linked to reduced menstrual pain and discomfort.

There are several reasons why maintaining a healthy weight can help reduce menstrual cramps. One reason is that excess weight can put additional stress on the pelvic region, which can worsen menstrual cramps. This added pressure can cause the uterus to contract more strongly, leading to more painful cramps.

Additionally, excess weight can lead to the production of more estrogen, which can cause the uterine lining to thicken. This thicker lining can lead to heavier and more painful periods. Conversely, losing weight can reduce estrogen levels and lead to lighter, less painful periods.

Research has also shown that maintaining a healthy weight can reduce inflammation in the body, which can help alleviate menstrual cramps. Chronic inflammation can exacerbate pain and discomfort, so reducing inflammation through a healthy diet and exercise can have a positive impact on menstrual cramps.

In addition to weight management, there are other lifestyle factors that can help reduce menstrual cramps. Regular exercise, for example, can help alleviate menstrual pain and discomfort by increasing blood flow and reducing inflammation. A healthy diet that is rich in fruits, vegetables, and whole grains can also help reduce inflammation and promote overall health.

It's important to note that while maintaining a healthy weight can have a positive impact on menstrual cramps, it's not a guarantee. Some women may experience menstrual pain and discomfort regardless of their weight. Additionally, there may be underlying medical conditions that contribute to menstrual cramps, such as endometriosis or fibroids. If you experience severe menstrual pain, it's important to talk to your healthcare provider to rule out any underlying medical issues.

In conclusion, maintaining a healthy weight can have a positive impact on menstrual cramps. By reducing excess weight, women can alleviate pressure on the pelvic region, reduce estrogen levels, and reduce inflammation. Additionally, other lifestyle factors such as exercise, diet, hydration, and stress management can help alleviate menstrual pain and discomfort. While weight management is important for overall health, it's important to remember that there are many factors that contribute to menstrual cramps and that every woman's experience is unique.

Notes

Avoiding Tobacco and Alcohol

While there are several factors that can contribute to menstrual cramps, avoiding tobacco and alcohol has been found to be linked to reduced severity of cramps.

Tobacco and Menstrual Cramps:

Studies have shown that smoking cigarettes can increase the severity of menstrual cramps. One study published in the Journal of Pediatric and Adolescent Gynecology found that women who smoked cigarettes had significantly worse menstrual cramps compared to non-smokers. The researchers believe that the chemicals in cigarettes can cause inflammation and reduce blood flow to the uterus, which can lead to more severe cramps.

Furthermore, smoking has been found to interfere with the body's ability to produce estrogen, a hormone that plays a key role in the menstrual cycle. This disruption can lead to irregular periods and worsen menstrual cramps. Therefore, quitting smoking or avoiding tobacco products can help reduce the severity of menstrual cramps.

Alcohol and Menstrual Cramps:
Alcohol consumption can also contribute to menstrual cramps. Research has shown that alcohol consumption can disrupt the hormonal balance in the body, leading to irregular periods and more severe menstrual cramps. Additionally, alcohol is known to cause dehydration, which can exacerbate cramps and lead to other menstrual symptoms, such as headaches and fatigue.

Moreover, alcohol consumption can cause the liver to work harder to metabolize the alcohol, leading to increased inflammation in the body. Inflammation can cause pain and discomfort, which can worsen menstrual cramps. Therefore, avoiding or limiting alcohol consumption can help reduce the severity of menstrual cramps.

Other Benefits of Avoiding Tobacco and Alcohol:

In addition to reducing menstrual cramps, avoiding tobacco and alcohol can have other benefits for women's reproductive health. For example, smoking has been linked to decreased fertility and an increased risk of miscarriage. Moreover, alcohol consumption during pregnancy can lead to fetal alcohol syndrome, which can cause lifelong physical and mental health problems for the child.

Furthermore, avoiding tobacco and alcohol can improve overall health and reduce the risk of other health problems, such as heart disease, stroke, and cancer.

Conclusion

In conclusion, avoiding tobacco and alcohol can help reduce the severity of menstrual cramps. Smoking and alcohol consumption can disrupt the hormonal balance in the body and lead to inflammation, which can exacerbate cramps and other menstrual symptoms. Quitting smoking or avoiding tobacco products and limiting alcohol consumption can also have other benefits for women's reproductive and overall health.

Notes

Getting Enough Sleep

While there are various treatments for menstrual cramps, one aspect that is often overlooked is the link between getting enough sleep and the severity of menstrual cramps.
Sleep plays a crucial role in the body's overall health and well-being, including hormonal regulation. Hormonal fluctuations are one of the primary causes of menstrual cramps, and sleep can help regulate these hormonal changes. When we sleep, our bodies release hormones such as melatonin, which helps regulate the body's circadian rhythm and sleep-wake cycle. Adequate sleep also helps to balance other hormones in the body, such as cortisol and insulin, which can affect menstrual cramps.

Studies have shown that there is a correlation between lack of sleep and increased menstrual pain. One study found that women who slept less than six hours per night had a higher likelihood of experiencing more severe menstrual cramps than women who slept for at least eight hours per night. This may be because of the way that sleep affects the body's pain response. Sleep deprivation can increase the body's sensitivity to pain, making menstrual cramps feel more severe.

In addition to affecting pain perception, sleep also plays a role in inflammation. Inflammation is a common cause of menstrual cramps, and getting enough sleep can help reduce inflammation in the body. Sleep deprivation has been linked to increased inflammation, which can make menstrual cramps worse.

Another way that sleep can affect menstrual cramps is through its impact on stress levels. Stress can exacerbate menstrual cramps by increasing muscle tension and inflammation in the body. Sleep plays a crucial role in reducing stress levels, and getting enough sleep can help mitigate the impact of stress on menstrual cramps.

To ensure that you are getting enough sleep to manage menstrual cramps, it is important to establish good sleep hygiene habits. This includes maintaining a consistent sleep schedule, avoiding caffeine and alcohol before bed, and creating a relaxing sleep environment. Practicing stress-reducing techniques such as meditation or yoga can also help improve sleep quality and reduce stress levels.

In conclusion, there is a clear link between getting enough sleep and the severity of menstrual cramps. Sleep plays a crucial role in regulating hormones, reducing inflammation, and managing stress, all of which can affect menstrual cramps. By prioritizing good sleep hygiene habits, women can reduce the severity of menstrual cramps and improve their overall menstrual health.

Notes

Maintaining Good Hygiene

Maintaining good hygiene is important for overall health, but it also plays a significant role in managing menstrual cramps. Menstrual cramps, also known as dysmenorrhea, are a common condition that affects many women during their menstrual cycle. They can range from mild discomfort to severe pain, and can be caused by a variety of factors, including hormonal imbalances, inflammation, and uterine contractions. While maintaining good hygiene may not eliminate menstrual cramps entirely, it can help to reduce their severity and frequency.

Here are some of the ways in which good hygiene can help to manage menstrual cramps:

Reduce the Risk of Infection: Poor hygiene can lead to infections, such as bacterial vaginosis or yeast infections, which can worsen menstrual cramps. By maintaining good hygiene practices, such as regularly washing the genital area and changing pads or tampons frequently, the risk of infection can be reduced.

Improve Menstrual Flow: Good hygiene practices can also help to improve menstrual flow, which can reduce cramping. By using tampons or menstrual cups, which allow for more efficient flow, and avoiding tight clothing or underwear, which can restrict blood flow, women can help to reduce cramping.

Relaxation and Stress Reduction: Good hygiene practices can also help to promote relaxation and reduce stress, which can exacerbate menstrual cramps. Taking a warm bath, practicing yoga or meditation, or simply taking time to relax and unwind can help to reduce cramping and promote overall well-being.

Reduced Inflammation: Good hygiene practices, such as consuming a healthy diet and avoiding processed foods, can also help to reduce inflammation, which is a common cause of menstrual cramps. Inflammation can be caused by a variety of factors, including poor diet, lack of exercise, and stress, and can be exacerbated by poor hygiene practices.

Preventing Toxic Shock Syndrome: Good hygiene practices can also help to prevent toxic shock syndrome, a rare but serious condition that can occur when bacteria enter the bloodstream. Toxic shock syndrome can be caused by the use of tampons, and can lead to symptoms such as fever, vomiting, and confusion. By using tampons correctly and changing them frequently, the risk of toxic shock syndrome can be reduced.

In conclusion, maintaining good hygiene is essential for overall health and can also help to manage menstrual cramps. By reducing the risk of infection, improving menstrual flow, promoting relaxation, reducing inflammation, and preventing toxic shock syndrome, good hygiene practices can help to reduce the severity and frequency of menstrual cramps. Women should consult with their healthcare provider to develop an individualized plan to manage their menstrual cramps.

Notes

Chapter 6: Alternative and Complementary Treatments

Chiropractic Care

While there are various treatments available to alleviate the pain and discomfort associated with menstrual cramps, some women may be interested in exploring alternative therapies, such as chiropractic care.

Chiropractic care is a non-invasive form of healthcare that focuses on the diagnosis and treatment of musculoskeletal disorders, particularly those related to the spine. Chiropractors use manual therapies, such as spinal manipulation, to help alleviate pain and improve function in the body.

The link between chiropractic care and menstrual cramps is based on the concept that misalignments or subluxations in the spine can interfere with the body's natural functions and lead to pain and discomfort. It is believed that correcting these misalignments through chiropractic adjustments can help reduce menstrual cramps and other symptoms associated with the menstrual cycle.

Here are some of the ways that chiropractic care can potentially help alleviate menstrual cramps:

Reducing Muscle Tension: Chiropractic adjustments can help reduce muscle tension in the pelvic area, which can help alleviate menstrual cramps. By targeting the nerves and muscles in the spine, chiropractors can help improve blood flow and reduce inflammation, which can further reduce pain and discomfort.

Improving Spinal Alignment: Misalignments in the spine can lead to nerve interference, which can cause a wide range of health issues, including menstrual cramps. By correcting these misalignments through chiropractic adjustments, chiropractors can help improve spinal alignment and reduce nerve interference, which can help alleviate menstrual cramps.

Enhancing Overall Well-being: Chiropractic care is focused on improving overall health and well-being, which can help reduce the severity and frequency of menstrual cramps. By addressing any underlying health issues and improving the body's ability to function optimally, chiropractic care can help reduce the discomfort associated with menstrual cramps.

It is important to note that while chiropractic care may be helpful in reducing menstrual cramps, it is not a cure-all solution. Women should always consult with their healthcare provider before seeking chiropractic care or any other form of alternative therapy.

In addition, chiropractic care may not be appropriate for all women, particularly those with certain medical conditions or those who are pregnant. It is important to discuss any potential risks and benefits of chiropractic care with a qualified healthcare provider before seeking treatment.

In conclusion, while more research is needed to fully understand the link between chiropractic care and menstrual cramps, there is evidence to suggest that chiropractic care may be a helpful adjunct therapy for women experiencing menstrual cramps. By addressing misalignments in the spine, reducing muscle tension, and improving overall well-being, chiropractic care can potentially help alleviate menstrual cramps and other symptoms associated with the menstrual cycle.

Notes

Homeopathy

Conventional treatments for menstrual cramps often include over-the-counter pain relievers, hormonal birth control, and other prescription medications. However, some women may prefer to explore alternative treatments, such as homeopathy, to alleviate their menstrual cramps.

This is a form of alternative medicine that uses highly diluted substances to stimulate the body's natural healing processes. It is based on the principle of "like cures like," meaning that a substance that can cause symptoms in a healthy person can also help alleviate those same symptoms in a sick person. Homeopathic remedies are derived from natural sources, such as plants, minerals, and animal products, and are chosen based on the individual's specific symptoms and overall health.

There are several homeopathic remedies that may be helpful for menstrual cramps. Below are some commonly used remedies and their indications:

Magnesia Phosphorica: This remedy is often used for cramping pain that is relieved by warmth, such as a heating pad or hot water bottle. The pain may be located in the lower abdomen or back, and may be accompanied by shooting pains or spasms.

Colocynthis: This remedy is often used for cramping pain that is relieved by bending over or applying pressure to the abdomen. The pain may be located in the lower abdomen or back, and may be accompanied by diarrhea or nausea.

Belladonna: This remedy is often used for sudden and intense cramping pain, especially if the pain is accompanied by a flushed face, dilated pupils, or a throbbing headache. The pain may be located in the lower abdomen or back, and may be worsened by movement or touch.

Cimicifuga: This remedy is often used for cramping pain that is accompanied by mood swings, irritability, or anxiety. The pain may be located in the lower abdomen or back, and may be accompanied by stiffness or soreness in the muscles.

Pulsatilla: This remedy is often used for cramping pain that is accompanied by a heavy or bloated feeling in the abdomen. The pain may be located in the lower abdomen or back, and may be worsened by warmth or pressure.

It is important to note that homeopathic remedies should always be chosen based on the individual's specific symptoms and overall health, and should only be taken under the guidance of a qualified homeopathic practitioner. While homeopathy is generally considered safe, it is important to seek medical attention if menstrual cramps are severe or accompanied by other symptoms, such as fever, heavy bleeding, or unusual discharge.

In conclusion, menstrual cramps can be a frustrating and painful experience for many women. While conventional treatments may be effective for some, others may prefer to explore alternative treatments, such as homeopathy. Homeopathic remedies may offer a safe and natural option for alleviating menstrual cramps, but it is important to choose remedies based on individual symptoms and to seek guidance from a qualified practitioner.

Notes

Ayurvedic Medicine

Ayurveda, the traditional medicine system of India, is a holistic approach to health and well-being. Ayurveda is based on the concept that every individual is unique and therefore requires personalized treatment. Ayurveda views menstrual cramps, also known as dysmenorrhea, as a symptom of an imbalance in the body. In Ayurveda, menstrual cramps are classified as a vata dosha disorder. Vata is one of the three doshas in Ayurveda, and it is associated with movement and change in the body. In this article, we will explore the link between Ayurvedic medicine and menstrual cramps.

Ayurvedic View of Menstrual Cramps:
In Ayurveda, menstrual cramps are seen as a result of an imbalance in the body's doshas. The imbalance may be caused by factors such as stress, poor diet, lack of exercise, or hormonal changes. Menstrual cramps are a sign that the body is trying to eliminate toxins and excess vata energy from the body. Ayurveda sees menstrual cramps as a natural process of cleansing and detoxifying the body.

Ayurvedic Treatment for Menstrual Cramps:
The treatment of menstrual cramps in Ayurveda involves balancing the vata dosha in the body. Ayurveda offers various remedies that can help alleviate menstrual cramps. Here are some of the Ayurvedic treatments for menstrual cramps:

Herbal Remedies:
Ayurveda recommends various herbal remedies to alleviate menstrual cramps. Some of the herbs used in Ayurveda include ginger, fennel, cumin, and coriander. These herbs have anti-inflammatory and analgesic properties that can help reduce the pain and inflammation associated with menstrual cramps.

Diet and Lifestyle Changes:
Ayurveda believes that a balanced diet and lifestyle can help reduce menstrual cramps. Ayurvedic experts recommend a diet that is rich in fruits, vegetables, whole grains, and lean proteins. They also recommend avoiding foods that are spicy, oily, or fried.

In addition to dietary changes, Ayurveda also recommends lifestyle changes such as getting regular exercise, practicing stress-reducing techniques such as yoga and meditation, and getting enough sleep.

Abhyanga:
Abhyanga is an Ayurvedic massage technique that involves the use of warm oils. This massage technique can help reduce pain and inflammation associated with menstrual cramps. The massage is typically done on the lower abdomen, lower back, and pelvic area.

Panchakarma
This is an Ayurvedic detoxification treatment that involves a series of therapies. Panchakarma can help eliminate toxins from the body, reduce inflammation, and improve circulation. This treatment can be effective in reducing menstrual cramps.

Ayurvedic Herbs:
Ayurvedic herbs such as Ashoka, Lodhra, and Shatavari are commonly used to alleviate menstrual cramps. These herbs can help regulate hormones, reduce inflammation, and improve circulation.

Conclusion:

Ayurveda offers a holistic approach to treating menstrual cramps. Ayurvedic remedies can help alleviate menstrual cramps by balancing the vata dosha in the body. Ayurvedic treatments such as herbal remedies, diet and lifestyle changes, massage, panchakarma, and Ayurvedic herbs can be effective in reducing menstrual cramps.

Notes

Naturopathic Medicine

Naturopathic medicine is a form of complementary and alternative medicine that emphasizes the use of natural remedies to support the body's inherent healing ability. Naturopathic medicine has gained popularity as a treatment option for menstrual cramps, a common issue experienced by women during their menstrual cycle. This comprehensive content will explore the link between naturopathic medicine and menstrual cramps.

Naturopathic medicine views menstrual cramps as a sign of an underlying imbalance in the body. The goal of naturopathic treatment for menstrual cramps is to address the root cause of the condition and provide symptomatic relief.

Here are some naturopathic treatments that can be helpful in managing menstrual cramps:

Herbal Medicine: Naturopathic medicine relies heavily on the use of herbal medicine to manage menstrual cramps. Some herbs, such as ginger and turmeric, have anti-inflammatory properties that can help reduce the severity of menstrual cramps. Other herbs, such as cramp bark and black cohosh, are believed to have muscle-relaxing properties that can help reduce the intensity of cramps.

Acupuncture: Acupuncture is a traditional Chinese medicine technique that involves inserting thin needles into specific points on the body to alleviate pain and discomfort. Research has shown that acupuncture can be an effective treatment for menstrual cramps.

Dietary changes: Naturopathic doctors recommend making dietary changes to help manage menstrual cramps. Foods that are rich in magnesium, such as leafy greens, nuts, and whole grains, can help reduce cramps. Omega-3 fatty acids found in fatty fish like salmon, mackerel, and sardines can also help reduce inflammation and alleviate cramps.

Exercise: Regular exercise can help reduce the severity of menstrual cramps. Naturopathic doctors may recommend gentle exercises such as yoga or walking to help manage cramps.

Stress management: Stress can exacerbate menstrual cramps, and naturopathic doctors may recommend stress management techniques such as meditation and deep breathing exercises to help manage cramps.

In addition to these naturopathic treatments, it is important to maintain good menstrual hygiene practices such as using sanitary pads, changing them regularly, and avoiding the use of tampons during the menstrual cycle.

In conclusion, naturopathic medicine offers a holistic approach to managing menstrual cramps. By addressing the underlying causes of the condition and providing symptomatic relief, naturopathic medicine can help women manage their menstrual cramps and improve their overall quality of life. However, it is essential to consult with a licensed naturopathic doctor before starting any naturopathic treatments to ensure that they are safe and effective for individual

Notes

Chapter 7: Conclusion

Recap of Menstrual Cramps and their Management

Menstrual cramps, also known as dysmenorrhea, are a common problem among women during their menstrual cycle. These cramps are caused by the contraction of the uterus as it sheds its lining during menstruation. Menstrual cramps can be mild to severe and can affect a woman's daily life. In this article, we will provide a comprehensive recap of menstrual cramps and their management.

Types of Menstrual Cramps

There are two types of menstrual cramps: primary dysmenorrhea and secondary dysmenorrhea.

Primary dysmenorrhea: This type of menstrual cramp is caused by the release of prostaglandins, which are hormone-like substances that cause the uterus to contract. Primary dysmenorrhea usually occurs in teenage girls and young women and is often accompanied by other symptoms such as nausea, diarrhea, and headache.

Secondary dysmenorrhea: This type of menstrual cramp is caused by an underlying medical condition such as endometriosis, uterine fibroids, or pelvic inflammatory disease. Secondary dysmenorrhea usually occurs in women who are in their 30s or 40s and is often accompanied by heavy bleeding and other symptoms such as fatigue and back pain.

Symptoms of Menstrual Cramps

The symptoms of menstrual cramps can vary from person to person, but the most common symptoms include:

Cramping in the lower abdomen or pelvis
Pain that radiates to the lower back and thighs
Nausea
Diarrhea
Headache
Fatigue
Management of Menstrual Cramps

Over-the-counter pain medication: Nonsteroidal anti-inflammatory drugs (NSAIDs) such as ibuprofen or naproxen can be effective in relieving menstrual cramps. These medications work by blocking the production of prostaglandins, which cause the uterus to contract. It is important to follow the recommended dosage and not exceed the daily limit.

Heat therapy: Applying a heating pad or hot water bottle to the lower abdomen can help to relieve menstrual cramps. The heat helps to relax the muscles and increase blood flow to the area.

Exercise: Regular exercise can help to reduce the severity of menstrual cramps. Exercise releases endorphins, which are natural painkillers, and can also improve blood flow to the pelvic area.

Relaxation techniques: Relaxation techniques such as deep breathing, meditation, and yoga can help to reduce stress and tension, which can worsen menstrual cramps.

Dietary changes: Making dietary changes such as reducing salt intake, increasing water consumption, and avoiding caffeine and alcohol can help to reduce the severity of menstrual cramps.

Prescription medication: If over-the-counter pain medication is not effective, a doctor may prescribe stronger pain medication or hormonal birth control to help manage menstrual cramps.

Surgery: In severe cases of secondary dysmenorrhea, surgery may be necessary to remove the underlying medical condition causing the menstrual cramps.

Conclusion

Menstrual cramps can be a painful and disruptive part of a woman's menstrual cycle. However, there are many management options available to help relieve the pain and discomfort associated with menstrual cramps. It is important to speak with a healthcare provider if menstrual cramps are interfering with daily life or if there are other concerning symptoms present. With the right management, menstrual cramps can be effectively controlled and managed.

Final Thoughts and Encouragement to seek help if needed.

Menstrual cramps are a common issue that many women experience during their menstrual cycle. These cramps, also known as dysmenorrhea, can range from mild discomfort to severe pain and can affect a woman's daily activities and quality of life. While menstrual cramps are a natural part of the menstrual cycle, there are ways to manage and alleviate the discomfort.

Firstly, it is essential to understand the causes of menstrual cramps. During the menstrual cycle, the uterus contracts to shed its lining, causing cramps. The hormone prostaglandin is responsible for these contractions and is produced in higher amounts during menstruation. High levels of prostaglandins can lead to more severe menstrual cramps.

There are several methods for managing menstrual cramps, both at home and with medical help. One effective way to manage menstrual cramps is by using over-the-counter pain relievers such as ibuprofen, naproxen, or acetaminophen. These medications can help alleviate the pain associated with menstrual cramps. Applying heat to the affected area, such as using a heating pad or taking a warm bath, can also help to alleviate pain and discomfort.

In addition to these home remedies, there are medical treatments available for more severe menstrual cramps. For example, hormonal birth control can help to regulate hormone levels and reduce the severity of menstrual cramps. In some cases, a doctor may prescribe prescription-strength pain relievers or prescribe medication to reduce prostaglandin production.

It is essential to seek medical help if menstrual cramps are interfering with daily activities or are unusually severe. Ignoring the symptoms can lead to more severe issues, such as endometriosis or pelvic inflammatory disease. Seeking medical attention can help to identify the underlying cause of menstrual cramps and provide more effective treatment.

It is also important to note that menstrual cramps are not a sign of weakness or an indication of inadequate strength. Many women experience menstrual cramps, and it is a natural part of the menstrual cycle. Seeking help or treatment for menstrual cramps is not something to be ashamed of or embarrassed about.

In conclusion, menstrual cramps are a common and natural part of the menstrual cycle. There are many ways to manage and alleviate the discomfort associated with menstrual cramps, both at home and with medical help. It is essential to seek medical attention if menstrual cramps are interfering with daily activities or are unusually severe. Remember that seeking help is not a sign of weakness, and there is no shame in seeking medical attention for menstrual cramps.

Additional Notes:

Explanation:

1. What are menstrual cramps, and what is their medical definition?

2. What causes menstrual cramps, and how do they occur?

3. What types of menstrual cramps are there, and how do they differ from each other?

4. How do menstrual cramps affect a woman's body, and what is the mechanism behind this?

Prevalence:

1. How common are menstrual cramps, and what percentage of women experience them?

2. Do menstrual cramps tend to occur more frequently in certain age groups or demographics?

3. Are there any factors that increase a woman's risk of experiencing menstrual cramps, such as lifestyle choices or medical conditions?

Myths:

1. Are menstrual cramps just "all in a woman's head," or is there a biological basis for their occurrence?

2. Do menstrual cramps go away once a woman gives birth, or do they persist?

3. Can menstrual cramps be completely cured, or is there no definitive treatment?

4. Are there any myths surrounding menstrual cramps that need to be debunked, such as certain home remedies or folk remedies that are ineffective or even harmful?

1. What are some of the most common misconceptions about menstrual cramps,
and how can they be corrected?

____

____

____

____

____

2. Are there any long-term health effects associated with menstrual cramps, such
as infertility or chronic pain?

____

____

____

____

____

____

3. Can menstrual cramps be a symptom of a more serious medical condition, and what are some signs that a woman should seek medical attention?

Chapter 2

Types of Menstrual Cramps:
1. What are the two types of menstrual cramps?

2. What is primary dysmenorrhea?

3. What is secondary dysmenorrhea?

4. How do the symptoms of primary and secondary dysmenorrhea differ?

Causes of Menstrual Cramps:

1. What causes menstrual cramps?

2. How does the uterus cause menstrual cramps?

3. How does hormonal imbalance cause menstrual cramps?

4. How does endometriosis cause menstrual cramps?

5. How does uterine fibroids cause menstrual cramps?

When to Seek Medical Help:

1. When should I seek medical help for menstrual cramps?

2. What are the warning signs that my menstrual cramps may be a more serious issue?

3. Can menstrual cramps be a sign of an underlying medical condition?

4. What tests may be done to diagnose the cause of my menstrual cramps?

5. How can I manage my menstrual cramps at home, and when should I see a doctor for further treatment?

Chapter 3

1. What dietary changes can be made to alleviate menstrual cramps?

2. How does regular exercise help in managing menstrual cramps?

3. Is heat therapy effective in managing menstrual cramps? If so, what are some methods that can be used?

4. Are there any herbal remedies that can help relieve menstrual cramps? If yes, what are they and how should they be consumed?

5. What is acupuncture, and how does it help with menstrual cramps?

6. Can massage help in reducing the severity of menstrual cramps? If so, what type of massage is recommended?

7. How long before menstrual cramps should one start incorporating these methods into their routine?

8. Are there any precautions that need to be taken before trying any of these methods?

9. How long does it typically take to see results from these methods?

____

____

____

____

10. Can these methods be used in conjunction with traditional medicine for menstrual cramps?

____

____

____

____

____

____

Chapter 4

1. Over-the-counter medications:

a. What over-the-counter medications are commonly used to manage menstrual cramps?

____

____

____

____

____

b. How do these medications work to alleviate menstrual cramps?

____

____

____

____

c. What are the potential side effects of over-the-counter medications used for menstrual cramps?

____

____

____

____

d. Can over-the-counter medications be used in combination with other treatments for menstrual cramps, such as hormonal birth control or surgical procedures?

2. Prescription medications:

a. What prescription medications are commonly used to manage menstrual cramps?

b. How do these medications work to alleviate menstrual cramps?

c. What are the potential side effects of prescription medications used for menstrual cramps?

d. Can prescription medications be used in combination with other treatments for menstrual cramps, such as hormonal birth control or surgical procedures?

3. Hormonal birth control:

a. How does hormonal birth control help manage menstrual cramps?

b. What types of hormonal birth control are commonly used for menstrual cramps?

____

____

____

____

c. What are the potential side effects of hormonal birth control used for menstrual cramps?

____

____

____

____

d. Can hormonal birth control be used in combination with other treatments for menstrual cramps, such as over-the-counter or prescription medications or surgical procedures?

____

____

____

____

4. Surgical procedures:

a. What surgical procedures are available for the management of menstrual cramps?

b. How do these surgical procedures work to alleviate menstrual cramps?

c. What are the potential risks and benefits of surgical procedures used for menstrual cramps?

d. Can surgical procedures be used in combination with other treatments for menstrual cramps, such as over-the-counter or prescription medications or hormonal birth control?

5. General questions:

a. What are the most effective treatments for menstrual cramps?

b. How do treatment options vary based on the severity of menstrual cramps?

c. When should a person see a healthcare provider for menstrual cramp management?

d. Are there any lifestyle changes or alternative therapies that can help alleviate menstrual cramps?

e. Can menstrual cramps be a sign of a more serious underlying condition?

Chapter 5

1. What are some strategies for maintaining a healthy weight that can help manage menstrual cramps?

2. How can avoiding alcohol and tobacco help with menstrual cramp management?

3. What role does getting enough sleep play in reducing menstrual cramps?

4. What are some good hygiene practices that can help with menstrual cramp management?

5. How can exercise help with menstrual cramp management?

6. Can certain dietary changes help manage menstrual cramps?

7. Are there any natural remedies that can be used to manage menstrual cramps?

8. How can stress management techniques like meditation or yoga help with menstrual cramp management?

9. What are some over-the-counter pain relievers that can be used for menstrual cramp management?

10. When should a person see a healthcare provider for menstrual cramp management?

Chapter 6

1. What is chiropractic medicine and how does it help in managing menstrual cramps?

2. How do chiropractic adjustments work to relieve menstrual cramps?

3. What are the potential risks or side effects associated with chiropractic treatment for menstrual cramps?

4. How does homeopathy work in managing menstrual cramps?

5. What homeopathic remedies are commonly used for menstrual cramp management?

6. What is Ayurvedic medicine and how does it help in managing menstrual cramps?

7. What are the commonly used Ayurvedic remedies for menstrual cramp management?

8. How does naturopathic medicine help in managing menstrual cramps?

9. What are some common naturopathic treatments for menstrual cramps?

10. Can these alternative medicine practices completely eliminate menstrual cramps?

11. How do these alternative medicine practices compare to traditional medical treatments for menstrual cramps in terms of effectiveness?

12. What is the evidence-based research on these alternative medicine practices
for menstrual cramp management?

13. Can these alternative medicine practices be used in conjunction with
traditional medical treatments for menstrual cramps?

14. What precautions should be taken when using these alternative medicine
practices for menstrual cramp management?

15. How can one find a qualified practitioner for these alternative medicine practices related to menstrual cramp management?